Heartfelt Health: Empowering Strategies for Managing Heart Disease and Stroke

Dr. Roseline Vasiyev PhD

STORY !!

Once upon a time, in a quiet suburban neighbourhood, lived Darren, a resilient and determined 67-year-old man. Darren had always been an active and health-conscious individual, cherishing his daily morning walks, tending to his garden, and relishing nutritious homemade meals. Despite his efforts, life had a surprise in store for him – a sudden stroke that forever altered the course of his journey.

One bright morning, as Darren embarked on his usual stroll through the neighbourhood park, he suddenly stumbled and fell to the ground. Panic and confusion gripped him as his speech slurred, and his limbs felt strangely heavy. Fortunately, a passerby noticed his distress and swiftly called for medical help. Within minutes, an ambulance arrived, rushing Darren to the nearby hospital.

The doctors diagnosed Darren with an ischemic stroke, a condition caused by a clot that had blocked a blood vessel in his brain. As he lay in the hospital bed, Darren's determination to reclaim his life burned stronger than ever. With the support of his family and the guidance of his medical team, he began the arduous process of rehabilitation.

Weeks turned into months as Darren underwent intensive physical therapy, speech therapy, and occupational therapy. Each session was a testament to his unwavering spirit, as he pushed himself to regain his strength, coordination, and communication skills. There were moments of frustration and exhaustion, but Darren's resolve never wavered.

During his recovery, Darren's doctors also identified underlying heart disease, which had contributed to his stroke. This revelation only fueled his determination to take charge of his health. He embraced a heart-healthy diet, carefully monitoring his sodium intake, reducing saturated fats, and incorporating a variety of fruits, vegetables, and whole grains into his meals.

With the guidance of his healthcare team, Darren established a personalised exercise routine that balanced his physical limitations with his desire for progress. He engaged in gentle cardiovascular exercises, strength training, and even took up yoga to enhance his flexibility and reduce stress.

But Darren's journey wasn't just about physical recovery; it was a holistic transformation. He delved into stress-relief techniques, incorporating mindfulness meditation and deep breathing exercises into his daily routine. He joined a local support group for stroke survivors, where he found camaraderie, shared experiences, and a sense of belonging that motivated him to persevere.

As months turned into years, Darren's dedication yielded remarkable results. He regained his ability to walk steadily, his speech became clearer, and his overall vitality was on the rise. With careful management of his heart disease through medication and lifestyle changes, his risk of future strokes diminished significantly.

Darren's story became an inspiration to his community and beyond. He started giving talks at local health fairs and senior centres, sharing his journey of overcoming stroke and managing heart disease. His message was clear: with determination, education, and a strong support system, one could not only survive but thrive after facing such health challenges.

Darren's remarkable tale serves as a reminder that resilience knows no age limits. With the right mindset and a willingness to adapt, even life's most unexpected twists can be met with courage and transformed into stories of triumph.

Introduction

Welcome to "Heartfelt Health: Empowering Strategies for Managing Heart Disease and Stroke." In the pages of this comprehensive guide, you will embark on a journey towards a healthier heart and a brighter future. Heart disease and stroke are formidable adversaries, affecting millions of lives worldwide and posing significant challenges to our well-being. However, armed with the right knowledge, strategies, and a commitment to change, you can take control of your cardiovascular health and enhance your quality of life.

In the following chapters, we will delve deep into the intricacies of heart disease and stroke, shedding light on their causes, risk factors, and the latest advancements in medical research. But this book goes beyond mere information – it is a manual of empowerment, providing you with actionable steps, expert insights, and practical advice to actively manage your condition and reduce your risk.

Our goal is not only to equip you with the tools you need but also to inspire you to embrace a heart-healthy lifestyle with enthusiasm and determination. You will discover that making positive changes doesn't have to be overwhelming; small, consistent adjustments can lead to remarkable transformations. From adopting heart-smart dietary habits and embracing regular physical activity to managing stress and cultivating a supportive network, you will find a wealth of guidance tailored to your unique needs.

Moreover, "Heartfelt Health" recognizes the vital role of collaboration between you and your healthcare team. We will explore the importance of effective communication, understanding medical treatments, and engaging in shared decision-making to ensure that you receive the best care possible. With the right information at your fingertips, you will be better prepared to make informed choices about your health and treatment options.

Throughout this book, you will encounter real-life stories of individuals who have navigated the challenges of heart disease and stroke. Their experiences serve as powerful reminders that you are not alone on this journey and that positive outcomes are achievable. By drawing inspiration from their achievements, you will find the motivation to persevere and make lasting changes that contribute to your overall well-being.

As you embark on this voyage of self-discovery and transformation, keep in mind that every step you take towards better heart health is a step towards a brighter future. "Heartfelt Health" is your compass, guiding you towards a life filled with vitality, joy, and longevity. So, let's embark on this transformative expedition together, as we uncover the path to managing heart disease and stroke with wisdom, courage, and a genuine commitment to a healthier heart.

<u>Focus 1</u>
<u>Focus 2</u>
<u>Focus 3</u>
<u>Focus 4</u>
<u>Focus 5</u>
<u>Focus 6</u>
<u>Focus 7</u>
<u>Focus 8</u>
<u>Focus 9</u>
<u>Focus 10</u>
<u>Focus 11</u>
<u>Focus 12</u>

Focus 1: Understanding Heart Disease and Stroke

Understanding the intricacies of heart disease and stroke is fundamental to embarking on a journey towards improved cardiovascular health. These conditions are complex and multifaceted, and delving deep into their causes, risk factors, and implications is crucial for making informed decisions and taking proactive steps to manage and prevent them.

1.1 Differentiating Between Heart Disease and Stroke:
Cardiovascular disease, also referred to as heart disease, is a broad term that

describes a number of conditions that have an impact on the structure and operation of the heart. These include coronary artery disease, heart failure, arrhythmias, and more.

Stroke: A stroke happens when the blood supply to the brain is interrupted, which causes brain cell damage. Ischemic strokes result from a blocked blood vessel, while hemorrhagic strokes involve bleeding within the brain.

1.2 Risk Factors and Causes:

Heart Disease: Risk factors for heart disease include high blood pressure, high cholesterol, smoking, diabetes, obesity, a sedentary lifestyle, and a family history of heart problems. Contributing causes involve a buildup of plaque in the arteries, inflammation, and damage to the heart muscle.

Stroke: Risk factors for stroke mirror those of heart disease, with additional factors such as atrial fibrillation (an irregular heart rhythm), previous strokes or transient ischemic attacks (TIAs), and certain blood disorders. Causes of strokes are often linked to blood clots or bleeding due to weakened blood vessels.

1.3 Genetic and Lifestyle Influences:

Genetic Factors: Family history can play a significant role in predisposing individuals to heart disease and stroke. Certain genetic traits and mutations may contribute to an increased risk, making it crucial for individuals with a family history to undergo regular screenings and adopt preventive measures.
Lifestyle Factors: Lifestyle choices, including diet, physical activity, smoking, and stress management, heavily impact heart health. Unhealthy habits can

exacerbate genetic predispositions, while adopting a heart-healthy lifestyle can mitigate risks.

1.4 Early Detection and Diagnosis:

Recognising Symptoms: It's critical to be aware of the indicators of heart disease and stroke. Chest pain, shortness of breath, fatigue, and palpitations are some signs of heart disease.Stroke symptoms often involve sudden numbness or weakness in the face, arm, or leg, confusion, trouble speaking or understanding speech, and severe headaches.
Seeking Medical Attention: Prompt medical attention is crucial when symptoms arise. Timely diagnosis through medical history, physical examinations, imaging tests, and blood tests can facilitate effective treatment and management strategies.

1.5 Lifestyle Modifications for Prevention:

Heart-Healthy Diet: Adopting a diet rich in fruits, vegetables, whole grains, lean proteins, and healthy fats can significantly reduce the risk of heart disease and stroke. Limiting salt, saturated fats, and added sugars is vital.

Physical activity: Regular exercise supports healthy cholesterol, blood pressure, and weight levels.

Engaging in aerobic activities, strength training, and flexibility exercises contributes to overall cardiovascular fitness.

Smoking Cessation: Quitting smoking is one of the most impactful steps individuals can take to improve heart health and reduce stroke risk.

Blood Pressure and Cholesterol Management: Monitoring and controlling blood pressure and cholesterol levels through medication and lifestyle adjustments are pivotal for prevention.

Understanding heart disease and stroke provides a solid foundation for taking charge of one's cardiovascular health. By comprehending the distinctions, risk factors, and lifestyle influences associated with these conditions, individuals can make informed choices, work closely with healthcare providers, and implement effective strategies to manage and prevent heart disease and stroke.

Focus 2: Empowering Lifestyle Changes for Heart Disease and Stroke Management

Empowering lifestyle changes are at the core of effectively managing heart disease and stroke. By adopting heart-healthy habits and making intentional choices, individuals can enhance their cardiovascular health, reduce the risk of complications, and improve their overall quality of life.

2.1 Heart-Healthy Diet Plans and Recipes:

Balanced Nutrition: A heart-healthy diet emphasises nutrient-dense foods, including fruits, vegetables, whole grains, lean proteins, and healthy fats. The

Mediterranean diet and the DASH (Dietary Approaches to Stop Hypertension) diet are examples of dietary patterns associated with cardiovascular benefits.

Portion Control: Monitoring portion sizes helps manage calorie intake and maintain a healthy weight, which is crucial for heart disease and stroke prevention.

Reading Labels: Learning to read food labels allows individuals to make informed choices about sodium, added sugars, and trans fats, which can negatively impact heart health.

Meal Planning: Planning meals ahead of time helps ensure a balanced and nutritious diet, reducing the likelihood of making unhealthy food choices.

2.2 Importance of Regular Physical Activity:

Aerobic Exercise: Engaging in aerobic activities such as walking, jogging, swimming, and cycling strengthens the heart and improves circulation. Plan for at least 150 minutes of moderate intensity aerobic exercise every week.

Strength Training: Incorporating strength training exercises enhances muscle mass, metabolism, and overall cardiovascular fitness. Resistance bands, free weights, and bodyweight exercises can be effective.

Flexibility and Balance: Activities like yoga and tai chi promote flexibility, balance, and relaxation, reducing the risk of falls and injuries.

2.3 Strategies for Managing Weight and Reducing Obesity-Related Risks:

Body Mass Index (BMI): Understanding BMI and its implications for heart health provides a baseline for weight management goals.

Healthy Weight Loss: Gradual weight loss through a combination of diet and exercise is sustainable and reduces the strain on the heart.

Behaviour Modification: Mindful eating, keeping a food journal, and identifying emotional triggers for overeating contribute to successful weight management.

2.4 Mind and Heart Connection:

Stress Reduction Techniques: Managing stress through techniques such as deep breathing, meditation, progressive muscle relaxation, and mindfulness can positively impact heart health.

Sleep Quality: Prioritising sufficient and restful sleep supports overall well-being and helps regulate blood pressure and stress hormones.

Social Support: Cultivating positive relationships and engaging in social activities contribute to emotional well-being and stress reduction.

2.5 Integrating Lifestyle Changes Into Daily Routine:

Gradual Progress: Implementing lifestyle changes gradually increases the likelihood of long-term success.
Setting Realistic Goals: Establishing achievable goals and tracking progress fosters a sense of accomplishment and motivation.
Creating a Supportive Environment: Surrounding oneself with individuals who encourage healthy habits and provide accountability enhances the likelihood of sustaining positive changes.

2.6 Long-Term Benefits and Ongoing Commitment:

Consistency: Maintaining heart-healthy habits over the long term is essential for sustained improvements in cardiovascular health.

Cardiovascular Benefits: Lifestyle changes can lead to reduced blood pressure, improved cholesterol levels, better blood sugar control, and enhanced overall heart function.

Quality of Life: By prioritising heart health, individuals experience increased energy, better mood, and a decreased risk of heart-related complications.

Empowering lifestyle changes require dedication and commitment, but the rewards in terms of improved heart health and overall well-being are immeasurable. By embracing a heart-healthy diet, staying physically active, managing stress, and making intentional choices, individuals can take control of their cardiovascular health, reduce the risk of heart disease and stroke, and pave the way for a fulfilling and vibrant life.

Focus 3: Mind and Heart Connection

Understanding the intricate interplay between the mind and heart is pivotal in managing heart disease and stroke. The relationship between psychological well-being and cardiovascular health is profound, and nurturing a positive connection between the two can lead to improved outcomes and a higher quality of life.

3.1 Managing Stress and Its Impact on Heart Health:

Stress and Cardiovascular Health: Chronic stress can contribute to high blood pressure, inflammation, and an increased risk of heart disease and stroke.

Stress Response: The body's "fight or flight" response triggers the release of stress hormones, which can adversely affect the heart and blood vessels.

Stress Management Techniques: Engaging in relaxation techniques such as deep breathing, meditation, guided imagery, and progressive muscle relaxation helps reduce stress and its impact on the heart.

3.2 Practising Mindfulness, Meditation, and Relaxation:

Mindfulness: Mindfulness involves being fully present in the moment and cultivating awareness of thoughts, emotions, and sensations without judgement.

Meditation: Regular meditation practices promote relaxation, reduce anxiety, and lower blood pressure, thereby benefiting heart health.

Relaxation Techniques: Techniques such as visualisation, guided imagery, and aromatherapy provide avenues for relaxation and stress relief.

3.3 The Psychological Aspects of Recovery after a Stroke:

Emotional Impact: A stroke can elicit a range of emotions, including fear, frustration, sadness, and anxiety.

Post-Stroke Depression: Post-stroke depression is common and can negatively affect recovery. Identifying symptoms and seeking appropriate treatment are crucial.

Cognitive Changes: Stroke survivors may experience cognitive changes, such as memory impairment and difficulty concentrating. Rehabilitation and cognitive therapies can aid in recovery.

3.4 Cultivating a Positive Mindset:

Optimism and Resilience: Cultivating optimism and resilience contributes to better cardiovascular health outcomes. A positive outlook can lead to healthier lifestyle choices and improved adherence to treatment plans.

Gratitude Practice: Practising gratitude enhances psychological well-being and fosters a sense of contentment, which positively impacts heart health.

Social Connections: Maintaining strong social connections provides emotional support, reduces feelings of isolation, and promotes heart-healthy behaviours.

3.5 Emotional Intelligence and Heart Health:

Emotional Awareness: Developing emotional intelligence involves recognizing and managing emotions effectively, which can contribute to reduced stress and improved heart health.

Healthy Coping Strategies: Individuals with high emotional intelligence are more likely to use healthy coping strategies, such as seeking social support and engaging in positive activities.

3.6 Incorporating Mind-Body Practices Into Daily Life:

Holistic Well-Being: Mind-body practices integrate physical, emotional, and mental well-being, promoting a holistic approach to heart health.

Regular Practice: Consistency is key; incorporating mindfulness, meditation, and relaxation techniques into daily routines enhances their effectiveness over time.

Professional Guidance: Seeking guidance from mental health professionals or joining support groups can provide valuable tools and strategies for enhancing the mind-heart connection.

Nurturing a strong mind-heart connection is not only beneficial for managing heart disease and stroke but also for promoting overall well-being. By managing stress, practising mindfulness, cultivating a positive mindset, and harnessing emotional intelligence, individuals can create a harmonious relationship between their mental and cardiovascular health. This synergy can lead to reduced risk factors, improved recovery, and a higher quality of life for those navigating the journey of heart health management.

Focus 4: Medication and Treatment Options

Understanding the diverse range of medication and treatment options available for heart disease and stroke is crucial for effective management, prevention, and recovery. Medical interventions, combined with lifestyle changes, can significantly enhance cardiovascular health and improve overall well-being.

4.1 An Overview of Medications for Heart Disease and Stroke Prevention:

Antihypertensive Medications: Drugs that lower blood pressure, such as diuretics, ACE inhibitors, beta-blockers, and calcium channel blockers, help reduce the risk of heart disease and stroke.

Cholesterol-Lowering Medications: Statins and other lipid-lowering medications aid in managing cholesterol levels and preventing atherosclerosis.

Antiplatelet Agents: Medications like aspirin and clopidogrel help prevent blood clot formation and reduce the risk of stroke in certain individuals.

4.2 Surgical Interventions and Procedures:

Coronary Angioplasty and Stent Placement: This procedure involves widening narrowed or blocked arteries using a balloon catheter and placing a stent to keep the artery open.

Coronary Artery Bypass Grafting (CABG): CABG surgery creates a new pathway for blood to flow around blocked coronary arteries, improving blood supply to the heart muscle.

Carotid Endarterectomy: This surgery removes plaque buildup from the carotid arteries to reduce the risk of stroke.

4.3   Integrating   Complementary Therapies with Medical Treatments:

Acupuncture: Acupuncture may help manage certain cardiovascular risk factors, such as high blood pressure and stress.

Herbal Supplements: Some herbal supplements, like garlic and hawthorn, have been studied for their potential cardiovascular benefits. Consultation with a healthcare provider is essential before using any supplements.

4.4 Personalized Treatment Plans and Shared Decision-Making:

Collaborating with Healthcare Providers: Open communication with healthcare professionals is crucial for creating a personalised treatment plan that aligns with an individual's needs, preferences, and medical history.

Shared Decision-Making: Engaging in shared decision-making allows patients to actively participate in choosing the most appropriate treatment options based on their values and goals.

4.5 Adherence to Medication Regimens:

Importance of Adherence: Consistently taking prescribed medications as directed by healthcare providers is essential for achieving optimal treatment outcomes.

Overcoming Barriers: Addressing challenges such as cost, side effects, and forgetfulness can help improve medication adherence.

Medication Reviews: Periodic reviews with healthcare providers ensure that treatment plans remain effective and appropriate over time.

4.6 Monitoring and Adjusting Treatment Plans:

Regular Check-Ups: Routine follow-up appointments with healthcare providers allow for the monitoring of treatment progress and adjustments as needed.
Lifestyle Modifications: Integrating lifestyle changes alongside medication treatments enhances their effectiveness and promotes overall heart health.
Understanding medication options, surgical interventions, and complementary therapies empowers individuals to make informed decisions about their heart disease and stroke management. By working closely with healthcare providers, adhering to treatment regimens, and participating in shared decision-making, individuals can optimise their treatment plans, reduce risk factors, and improve their cardiovascular health and quality of life.

Focus 5: Shared Decision-Making and Communicating with Healthcare Providers

Effective communication and shared decision-making between patients and healthcare providers are cornerstones of successful heart disease and stroke management. Collaborative interactions empower individuals to actively participate in their care, make informed choices, and achieve optimal outcomes.

5.1 Building a Strong Patient-Doctor Relationship:

Open Communication: Establishing clear and open lines of communication with healthcare providers fosters trust, mutual understanding, and effective collaboration.

Patient-Centred Care: Patient-centred care places the individual's preferences, values, and goals at the forefront of treatment planning and decision-making.

5.2 Understanding Treatment Options and Making Informed Choices:

Education: Healthcare providers should provide comprehensive information about available treatment options, their benefits, risks, and potential outcomes.

Informed Consent: Informed consent involves ensuring that patients understand the proposed treatments, potential alternatives, and associated risks before making decisions.

5.3 Navigating the Healthcare System Effectively:

Coordination of Care: Healthcare providers play a crucial role in coordinating care among various specialists, ensuring that treatments align and information is shared.

Advocacy: Patients and their caregivers should advocate for their needs and preferences within the healthcare system to receive optimal care.

5.4 Engaging in Shared Decision-Making:

Collaborative Discussions: Shared decision-making involves meaningful discussions between patients and healthcare providers, considering medical evidence, personal values, and preferences.

Decision Aids: Decision aids, such as written materials or interactive tools, help patients understand treatment options and potential outcomes.

5.5 Ensuring Cultural Sensitivity and Health Literacy:

Cultural Competency: Healthcare providers should be sensitive to patients' cultural backgrounds, beliefs, and values to ensure that care is culturally appropriate.

Health Literacy: Clear communication in plain language ensures that patients understand medical information and can actively participate in decisions.

5.6 Obtaining Second Opinions:

Seek Additional Perspectives: Obtaining a second opinion from another qualified healthcare provider can provide valuable insights and options before making treatment decisions.

Respectful Approach: Seeking a second opinion is a normal part of the healthcare process and should be done in a respectful manner.

5.7 Adhering to Treatment Plans and Follow-Up:

Treatment Adherence: Following treatment plans as prescribed is essential for achieving desired outcomes. Patients and providers should work together to address barriers to adherence.

Regular Follow-Up: Scheduled follow-up appointments allow healthcare providers to monitor progress, adjust treatments as needed, and address any concerns.

5.8 Empowering Self-Advocacy:

Gathering Information: Patients should actively seek information about their condition, treatment options, and potential side effects to make informed decisions.

Asking Questions: Asking questions during appointments clarifies doubts, provides clarity on treatment plans, and facilitates shared decision-making.

Shared decision-making transforms the patient-provider relationship into a partnership where both parties work collaboratively to achieve the best possible outcomes. By engaging in open communication, understanding treatment options, advocating for their needs, and actively participating in their care, individuals can navigate the complexities of heart disease and stroke management with confidence and empowerment.

Focus 6: Support Systems and Coping Strategies

Building a robust support system and developing effective coping strategies are essential components of successfully navigating the challenges posed by heart disease and stroke. These elements provide emotional reinforcement, practical assistance, and the resilience needed for managing the physical and psychological aspects of these conditions.

6.1 Joining Support Groups for Stroke Survivors and Heart Disease Patients:

Emotional Connection: Support groups offer a space for individuals to connect with others who share similar experiences, fostering a sense of belonging and understanding.

Shared Knowledge: Participants can exchange information, insights, and strategies for managing daily life, treatment, and recovery.

Coping Skills: Support groups provide an avenue for learning effective coping skills, enhancing emotional well-being, and reducing feelings of isolation.

6.2 Coping with the Emotional Impact of a Health Crisis:

Acknowledging Emotions: Recognizing and acknowledging feelings of fear, anxiety, sadness, and frustration is an important step in the coping process.

Emotional Expression: Engaging in healthy emotional expression through journaling, creative arts, or talking with loved ones can alleviate emotional distress.

Professional Counselling: Seeking the assistance of mental health professionals can provide specialised guidance in coping with the emotional challenges of heart disease and stroke.

6.3 Engaging Family and Friends in the Recovery Process:

Building a Supportive Network: Involving family and friends in the recovery journey provides practical assistance, emotional support, and encouragement.

Communication: Open and honest communication with loved ones ensures that they understand the challenges and can provide appropriate assistance.

Education: Providing information to family and friends about the conditions, treatments, and lifestyle changes helps them become effective supporters.

6.4 Managing Stress and Finding Balance:

Stress-Reduction Techniques: Engaging in stress-relief activities such as meditation, yoga, deep breathing, and mindfulness helps manage stress levels.

Time Management: Prioritising tasks, setting realistic goals, and allowing time for relaxation contribute to a balanced lifestyle.

Seeking Professional Help: If stress becomes overwhelming, consulting mental health professionals can provide strategies for stress management.

6.5 Finding Meaning and Purpose:

Reevaluating Priorities: A health crisis often prompts individuals to reflect on their values and priorities, leading to positive lifestyle changes.

Engaging in Meaningful Activities: Pursuing hobbies, interests, and volunteer work can foster a sense of purpose and enhance emotional well-being.

6.6 Celebrating Achievements and Milestones:

Recognizing Progress: Celebrating even small achievements in recovery and lifestyle changes reinforces motivation and boosts self-esteem.

Supportive Environment: Sharing successes with loved ones and support groups generates encouragement and positive reinforcement.

6.7 Fostering Resilience and Embracing a Positive Outlook:

Resilience Building: Developing resilience involves adapting to challenges, bouncing back from setbacks, and maintaining a positive attitude.

Cognitive Reframing: Reframing negative thoughts into more positive and adaptive perspectives promotes emotional well-being.

Self-Compassion: Treating oneself with kindness and self-compassion in the face of challenges enhances emotional resilience.

Building a strong support system, utilising coping strategies, and fostering emotional resilience are vital components of managing heart disease and stroke. By engaging with support groups, seeking emotional support from loved ones, and developing effective coping mechanisms, individuals can navigate the emotional complexities of these conditions with greater confidence, strength, and a sense of purpose.

Focus 7: Preventing Secondary Strokes and Heart Events

Preventing secondary strokes and heart events is a critical aspect of managing heart disease and stroke. By understanding warning signs, adopting preventive measures, and making necessary lifestyle changes, individuals can significantly reduce the risk of recurrence and enhance their long-term cardiovascular health.

7.1 Identifying Warning Signs and Symptoms:

Stroke Warning Signs: Recognizing sudden numbness or weakness in the face, arm, or leg, confusion, trouble speaking or understanding speech, severe headaches, and vision problems can prompt immediate medical attention. Heart Attack Symptoms: Symptoms such as chest pain or discomfort, shortness of breath, nausea, lightheadedness, and pain or discomfort in the arms, back, neck, or jaw warrant urgent medical evaluation.

7.2 Reducing the Risk of Recurrent Strokes and Heart Events:

Medication Adherence: Consistently taking prescribed medications, such as antiplatelet agents and anticoagulants, can help prevent blood clot formation and reduce the risk of secondary strokes.
Blood Pressure Management: Monitoring and controlling blood pressure through lifestyle changes and medication adherence significantly reduces the risk of recurrent strokes and heart events.
Cholesterol Control: Managing cholesterol levels with medication and

dietary modifications decreases the likelihood of a subsequent heart event.

7.3   Long-Term   Strategies   for Maintaining Cardiovascular Health:

Heart-Healthy Lifestyle: Adhering to a heart-healthy diet, engaging in regular physical activity, and managing stress are fundamental for preventing secondary strokes and heart events.

Smoking Cessation: Quitting smoking and avoiding exposure to secondhand smoke dramatically lower the risk of recurrent cardiovascular events.

Diabetes Management: Maintaining optimal blood sugar levels through medication and lifestyle changes is crucial for preventing complications and secondary events.

7.4 Engaging in Regular Medical Check-Ups:

Monitoring Health: Regular medical appointments allow healthcare providers to monitor blood pressure, cholesterol levels, and overall cardiovascular health.
Early Detection: Detecting changes in health status or risk factors early enables prompt intervention and adjustments to treatment plans.

7.5 Implementing Lifestyle Changes for Long-Term Prevention:

Gradual Progress: Implementing lifestyle changes gradually increases the likelihood of sustained adherence and long-term success.
Customised Plans: Working with healthcare providers to develop personalised prevention plans ensures that strategies align with individual needs and preferences.

7.6 Psychological Well-Being and Secondary Prevention:

Emotional Resilience: Emotional well-being plays a role in preventing secondary strokes and heart events. Mind-Body Practices: Engaging in mindfulness, meditation, and relaxation techniques supports psychological health and reduces the risk of complications.

7.7 Advocating for Heart Health:

Public Awareness: Advocating for heart health within the community promotes awareness, encourages healthy lifestyle choices, and supports early intervention. Risk Education: Educating family, friends, and peers about the importance of recognizing warning signs and seeking medical attention can save lives.

Preventing secondary strokes and heart events requires a multifaceted approach that encompasses medical adherence, lifestyle modifications, regular check-ups, and psychological well-being. By being proactive, staying informed, and taking appropriate preventive measures, individuals can significantly reduce the risk of recurrence and contribute to a future of improved cardiovascular health and well-being.

Focus 8: Adapting to Lifestyle Changes

Adapting to lifestyle changes is a transformative process that lies at the heart of effectively managing heart disease and stroke. Embracing a new way of living, while navigating challenges and setbacks, empowers individuals to take control of their health, foster resilience, and achieve lasting well-being.

8.1 Overcoming Challenges and Setbacks:

Mindset Shift: Embracing a growth mindset, characterised by adaptability and perseverance, enables individuals to view challenges as opportunities for learning and growth.

Resilience Building: Developing resilience involves bouncing back from setbacks, maintaining a positive attitude, and cultivating coping skills to navigate obstacles.

8.2 Incorporating Modifications into Daily Routines:

Gradual Integration: Introducing lifestyle changes gradually increases the likelihood of successful adaptation and long-term adherence.

Sustainable Choices: Focusing on sustainable changes ensures that modifications become integrated parts of daily life.

8.3 Support Systems and Motivation:

Family and Friends: Involving loved ones as sources of encouragement, accountability, and practical assistance reinforces motivation.

Support Groups: Connecting with support groups provides a community of individuals facing similar challenges, fostering camaraderie and shared strategies.

8.4 Strategies for Sustained Success:

Setting Realistic Goals: Establishing achievable goals encourages a sense of accomplishment and bolsters motivation. Monitoring Progress: Tracking progress through journals, apps, or wearable devices provides visual evidence of success and areas for improvement.

8.5 Celebrating Milestones and Achievements:

Self-Recognition: Acknowledging and celebrating even small milestones reinforces motivation and self-esteem. Social Celebration: Sharing achievements with loved ones and support networks generates positive reinforcement and encouragement.

8.6 Fostering a Positive Relationship with Change:

Embracing Change: Cultivating a positive attitude towards change allows individuals to adapt more readily and view it as an opportunity for growth.

Flexibility: Being open to adjustments and modifications in the face of changing circumstances promotes adaptability.

8.7 Integrating Self-Care into Daily Life:

Prioritising Self-Care: Engaging in self-care practices, such as relaxation, hobbies, and mindfulness, promotes emotional well-being and resilience.

Mind-Body Connection: Recognizing the interconnectedness of physical and mental health encourages holistic self-care.

8.8 Seeking Professional Guidance and Adjustments:

Healthcare Provider Collaboration: Regular check-ups and consultations with healthcare professionals ensure that treatment plans and lifestyle changes remain aligned with health goals.

Modifications Over Time: Adapting lifestyle changes as health needs evolve ensures that strategies remain effective and relevant.

Adapting to lifestyle changes involves embracing transformation, cultivating resilience, and nurturing a positive relationship with change. By approaching challenges with a growth mindset, seeking support, and celebrating achievements, individuals can successfully integrate heart-healthy habits into their lives, contributing to improved cardiovascular health, enhanced well-being, and a brighter future.

Focus 9: Healthy Aging and Longevity

Navigating heart disease and stroke management in the context of healthy ageing is a dynamic and essential aspect of promoting longevity and maintaining a high quality of life. As individuals age, addressing cardiovascular health becomes increasingly important, and proactive measures can contribute to vitality and well-being in the later stages of life.

9.1 Addressing Heart Health Concerns in the Aging Population:

Age-Related Changes: Understanding the natural changes that occur in the cardiovascular system with age enables individuals to proactively address potential issues.

Prevention in Aging: Embracing heart-healthy habits earlier in life and continuing them as one ages can reduce the risk of heart disease and stroke.

9.2 Strategies for Maintaining Independence and Vitality:

Physical Activity: Engaging in regular exercise, tailored to individual capabilities, supports cardiovascular health, muscle strength, and mobility.

Fall Prevention: Incorporating balance exercises and home safety measures reduces the risk of falls and related injuries.

9.3 Creating a Fulfilling and Heart-Healthy Lifestyle in Senior Years:

Nutritional Considerations: Prioritising nutrient-rich foods, managing portion sizes, and staying hydrated contribute to heart health and overall well-being.

Social Engagement: Maintaining social connections, participating in activities, and pursuing interests promote emotional health and cognitive vitality.

9.4 Managing Age-Related Conditions:

Hypertension Management: Regular blood pressure monitoring and adherence to medication, if prescribed, play a vital role in preventing complications.

Diabetes Care: Managing blood sugar levels through medication, diet, and lifestyle changes reduces the risk of cardiovascular complications.

9.5 Cognitive Health and Heart-Brain Connection:

Brain Health: Adopting heart-healthy habits, such as a balanced diet and physical activity, positively impacts cognitive health and reduces the risk of cognitive decline.

9.6 Embracing Preventive Measures for Longevity:

Regular Check-Ups: Consistent medical check-ups and screenings enable early detection and management of heart-related issues.

Proactive Lifestyle Choices: Continuing to engage in heart-healthy habits, even in later years, contributes to overall well-being and longevity.

9.7 Emotional Resilience and Well-Being:

Coping with Loss: Addressing grief, loss, and life transitions through support networks and coping strategies enhances emotional resilience.

Positive Ageing Mindset: Cultivating a positive perspective on ageing fosters emotional well-being and adaptive coping.

9.8 Legacy and Contribution:

Volunteering and Community Involvement: Contributing to the community through volunteering and sharing wisdom supports a sense of purpose and fulfilment.

Passing Down Knowledge: Sharing experiences and lessons learned with younger generations contributes to family legacy and well-being.

Promoting healthy ageing and longevity involves a holistic approach that encompasses physical, emotional, and cognitive well-being. By proactively addressing cardiovascular health, embracing preventive measures, nurturing emotional resilience, and maintaining an active and engaged lifestyle, individuals can age gracefully, enhance their quality of life, and celebrate the journey of healthy ageing.

Focus 10: Inspiring Success Stories

Here are five inspiring success stories of individuals who effectively managed heart disease and stroke, showcasing resilience, determination, and the power of positive change:

Arnold's Active Golden Years:
After surviving a stroke in his late 60s, Arnold refused to let his condition define him. He embraced a heart-healthy lifestyle, committing to daily walks, engaging in water aerobics, and adopting a Mediterranean diet. Arnold's dedication not only improved his cardiovascular health but also inspired

his peers in the senior community to join him in pursuing active, vibrant lives.

Grace's Journey to Recovery:
Grace, a stroke survivor, experienced challenges in regaining her speech and mobility. With unwavering determination, she immersed herself in speech therapy, physical rehabilitation, and meditation. Through her resilience and strong support system, Grace made remarkable progress, relearning to speak and walk independently. Her story highlights the transformative power of perseverance.

Daniel's Lifestyle Transformation:
Diagnosed with heart disease in his early 40s, Daniel chose to take charge of his health. He embraced a plant-based diet, committed to regular exercise, and managed stress through meditation and yoga. Over time, he lost weight, reduced

his cholesterol levels, and improved his heart function. Daniel's journey demonstrates how significant lifestyle changes can lead to remarkable improvements in cardiovascular health.

Emily's Advocacy for Heart Health:
After experiencing a heart attack in her 50s, Emily became a passionate advocate for heart health awareness. She established a support group for women with heart disease, organised community events, and partnered with healthcare providers to offer educational workshops. Emily's efforts empowered countless individuals to prioritise heart health, leading to a healthier community.

Victor's Resilience in the Face of Adversity:
Victor faced a dual challenge of managing heart disease and recovering from a stroke. Despite setbacks, he embraced

physical therapy, adapted his home for safety, and engaged in cognitive exercises. Victor's determination and support from his family led to a remarkable recovery, allowing him to regain his independence and enjoy a fulfilling life.

These success stories serve as testament to the transformative potential of managing heart disease and stroke. Through determination, support, and a commitment to positive change, these individuals not only improved their own cardiovascular health but also inspired others to embark on their own journeys toward well-being and vitality.

Focus 11: Future Trends in Heart Disease and Stroke Management

The landscape of heart disease and stroke management is continually evolving as scientific advancements, technological innovations, and shifts in healthcare paradigms shape the way these conditions are understood, prevented, diagnosed, and treated. Exploring future trends in this field provides insight into the potential directions that cardiovascular care may take, offering promising avenues for improved outcomes and enhanced patient well-being.

11.1 Precision Medicine and Personalised Treatments:

Genomic Insights: Advances in genetic research enable the identification of individualised genetic factors contributing to heart disease and stroke risk, facilitating tailored treatment approaches.

Biomarker-Based Approaches: Utilising specific biomarkers to guide treatment decisions enhances precision in diagnosing and managing cardiovascular conditions.

11.2   Telemedicine   and   Remote Monitoring:

Virtual Care: Telemedicine platforms enable remote consultations, monitoring, and follow-up care, providing convenient access to healthcare professionals and reducing barriers to regular check-ups.

Wearable Technology: Wearable devices equipped with sensors can track vital signs, heart rhythms, and activity levels, empowering patients to actively manage their cardiovascular health.

11.3 Artificial Intelligence (AI) and Machine Learning:

Data Analysis: AI algorithms can analyse vast amounts of medical data to identify patterns, predict risk factors, and assist in early diagnosis and treatment planning.

Predictive Models: Machine learning models can forecast individualised heart disease and stroke risks, enabling proactive interventions and preventive strategies.

11.4 Targeted Therapies and Drug Development:

Novel Drug Classes: Emerging medications that target specific pathways implicated in heart disease and stroke offer potential for more effective and tailored treatments.

Gene Editing: Gene editing technologies may hold promise for correcting genetic mutations associated with cardiovascular conditions.

11.5 Regenerative Medicine and Stem Cell Therapy:

Tissue Regeneration: Stem cell therapies and regenerative approaches aim to repair damaged heart tissue and restore function, potentially revolutionising post-heart attack recovery.

Vascular Regrowth: Innovative techniques could stimulate the growth of new blood vessels, enhancing circulation and reducing the risk of ischemic events.

11.6 Behavioral Interventions and Digital Health:

Behavior Modification Apps: Digital platforms offer interactive tools for promoting healthy lifestyles, supporting individuals in adopting and sustaining heart-healthy behaviours.

Gamification: Gamified health apps engage users in goal-setting, tracking, and reward systems, promoting adherence to medication regimens and exercise routines.

11.7 Integrative Approaches to Mental and Emotional Well-Being:

Mind-Body Interventions: Holistic therapies such as mindfulness, meditation, and yoga are increasingly integrated into cardiovascular care to manage stress and improve emotional health.

Mental Health Integration: Recognizing the link between psychological well-being and cardiovascular health, healthcare systems prioritise mental health support for patients with heart disease and stroke.

Focus 12: Taking Charge of Your Heart Health

Taking charge of your heart health is a proactive and empowering approach to managing heart disease and stroke. By creating a personalised heart health plan, setting achievable goals, tracking progress, and celebrating milestones, individuals can navigate their journey with intention, determination, and a sense of accomplishment.

12.1 Creating a Personalized Heart Health Plan:

Assessment: Begin by assessing your current health status, including medical history, risk factors, and any existing conditions.

Consulting Healthcare Professionals: Collaborate with healthcare providers to tailor a heart health plan that addresses your specific needs, preferences, and goals.

Lifestyle Modifications: Incorporate recommended lifestyle changes, such as dietary adjustments, regular physical activity, stress management, and smoking cessation, into your plan.

12.2 Setting Achievable Goals:

Specific and Realistic: Define clear and realistic goals that align with your heart health objectives. For example, aim to walk 30 minutes a day, reduce sodium intake, or achieve a specific weight loss target.

Small Steps: Break down large goals into smaller, manageable steps to avoid feeling overwhelmed and enhance your chances of success.

SMART Goals: Apply the SMART (Specific, Measurable, Achievable, Relevant, Time-bound) framework to ensure that your goals are well-defined and achievable.

12.3 Tracking Progress:

Record Keeping: Maintain a journal, digital app, or tracking sheet to document your progress. Record relevant information, such as physical activity, dietary choices, medication adherence, and vital signs.

Regular Assessments: Schedule periodic assessments with your healthcare provider to monitor changes in cholesterol levels, blood pressure, weight, and other relevant markers.

Visual Motivation: Visual representations of your progress, such as charts or graphs, can provide a tangible sense of accomplishment and motivation.

12.4 Celebrating Milestones and Maintaining Motivation:

Recognizing Achievements: Acknowledge and celebrate even the smallest accomplishments along your heart health journey.

Reward System: Implement a reward system to treat yourself for reaching milestones. Rewards can be non-food related, such as enjoying a spa day, buying a new book, or spending quality time with loved ones.

Social Support: Share your achievements with friends, family, or support groups. Their encouragement and positive reinforcement can boost motivation.

12.5 Adapting and Refining Your Plan:

Flexibility: Recognize that progress is not always linear. Be adaptable and willing to adjust your plan based on new information, changing circumstances, and feedback from healthcare professionals.

Continuous Learning: Stay informed about heart health, new research, and emerging strategies. This knowledge empowers you to make informed decisions about your plan.

12.6 Cultivating Long-Term Habits:

Consistency: Consistently practising heart-healthy habits over time is key to achieving lasting improvements in cardiovascular health.

Mindful Choices: Incorporate mindfulness into your decision-making process, considering how your choices impact your overall well-being.

Life-Long Commitment: Taking charge of your heart health is a lifelong commitment. Embrace the journey as an opportunity to prioritise your well-being and longevity.

By creating a personalised heart health plan, setting achievable goals, tracking progress, and celebrating milestones, you are actively participating in your health and well-being. This approach empowers you to navigate heart disease and stroke management with purpose, resilience, and a greater sense of control over your cardiovascular health journey.